Miracle Essential Oils
25 Smellgoods To Make a Handmade Soap & Skincare

I0408438

Table of content

Introduction

There you are, standing in the store, and hoping to find something that is going to work for your dry, itchy skin. It always happens this time of year. It seems as soon as the air starts to get cooler, your skin starts to burn as it dries and starts to crack.

You want relief, but it can be hard to always have that lotion around, or to have to always stop and get lotion on, but then have to wait for it to dry before you can get back to your day. Of course, once it does dry, you are left with the problem once again.

If only there was a skin care product you could use that would solve your problem. Something that would take care of your dry skin and pamper you like you deserve, without costing and arm and a leg to do it. You know if you want the best of the best, you are going to have to make it yourself, but who has the time... or money... to get all the things you need to make your own soap?

Who wants to have those dangerous products sitting around the house, and who wants to have to worry about the kids when you finally do have time to make the soap? No, there has got to be an easier way.

After all, you see so many soaps online... so many soaps that busy people just like you have made. Soaps that are perfect for what you need, but not filled with chemicals you don't want on your body.

How do they do it? How do they get those wonderful soaps? Can you make them yourself? Isn't soap supposed to be hard to make?

If you have ever looked into making your own soap, odds are you were a little dismayed. There are so many things they say you need to get the job done, and so many things you don't want to have around your kids. But thankfully, there is a way around it, and you have found that way in this book.

I am going to show you how to make your own soap the easy way, and end up with the product you are looking for. I am going to show you exactly what you need to do to get the soap you have been dreaming of, while saving money and keeping your kids safe.

I am going to show you just what you need to have it all, and just what you have been missing all this time. I am going to unlock the door to complete pampering.

All you have to do is walk inside.

So get ready, your oasis awaits.

Chapter 1 – The Best of the Basics

Sometimes the best things come in the most simple of packages...

The Guava Goddess

What you will need:

10 drops grapefruit oil

5 drops lavender oil

5 drops orange oil

2 teaspoons coconut oil

½ teaspoon almond oil

1 bar all natural Ivory soap

Craft knife

Parchment paper

Directions:

Soften the bar of soap slight in the microwave. Cut into smaller pieces, and add to a pan on the stove with the coconut and almond oil.

Turn on to medium high heat, and stir often. Let the bar of soap completely melt, and once it has, add in all your essential oils.

Blend well, then remove from heat. Let the mix cool for a while. Stir every few minutes, and once it's cool enough to touch, roll out onto the parchment paper. Use your hands to form into a ball (carefully, you don't want to burn yourself), or use molds.

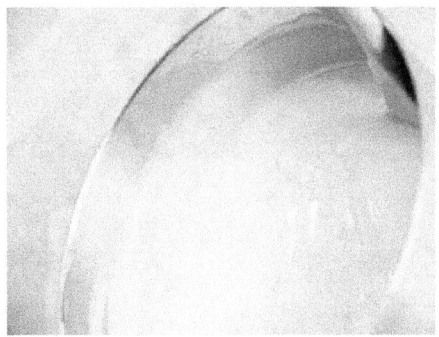

Let set up for 24 hours, and your handmade soap is done.

Petals and Princesses

What you will need:

10 drops rose oil

10 drops lavender oil

15 drops hibiscus oil

2 teaspoons coconut oil

½ teaspoon almond oil

1 bar all natural Ivory soap

Craft knife

Parchment paper

Directions:

Soften the bar of soap slight in the microwave. Cut into smaller pieces, and add to a pan on the stove with the coconut and almond oil.

Turn on to medium high heat, and stir often. Let the bar of soap completely melt, and once it has, add in all your essential oils.

Blend well, then remove from heat. Let the mix cool for a while. Stir every few minutes, and once it's cool enough to touch, roll out onto the parchment paper. Use your hands to form into a ball (carefully, you don't want to burn yourself), or use molds.

Let set up for 24 hours, and your handmade soap is done.

The Happy Bar

What you will need:

10 drops rose oil

15 drops plumeria aromatherapy oil

5 drops tea tree oil

2 teaspoons coconut oil

½ teaspoon almond oil

1 bar all natural Ivory soap

Craft knife

Parchment paper

Directions:

Soften the bar of soap slight in the microwave. Cut into smaller pieces, and add to a pan on the stove with the coconut and almond oil.

Turn on to medium high heat, and stir often. Let the bar of soap completely melt, and once it has, add in all your essential oils.

Blend well, then remove from heat. Let the mix cool for a while. Stir every few minutes, and once it's cool enough to touch, roll out onto the parchment paper. Use your hands to form into a ball (carefully, you don't want to burn yourself), or use molds.

Let set up for 24 hours, and your handmade soap is done.

Elegant Suds

What you will need:

12 drops myrrh oil

12 drops rosewood oil

5 drops cardamom oil

2 teaspoons coconut oil

½ teaspoon almond oil

1 bar all natural Ivory soap

Craft knife

Parchment paper

Directions:

Soften the bar of soap slight in the microwave. Cut into smaller pieces, and add to a pan on the stove with the coconut and almond oil.

Turn on to medium high heat, and stir often. Let the bar of soap completely melt, and once it has, add in all your essential oils.

Blend well, then remove from heat. Let the mix cool for a while. Stir every few minutes, and once it's cool enough to touch, roll out onto the parchment paper. Use your hands to form into a ball (carefully, you don't want to burn yourself), or use molds.

Let set up for 24 hours, and your handmade soap is done.

Silky Heaven

What you will need:

10 drops myrrh oil

15 drops jasmine oil

10 drops geranium oil

2 teaspoons coconut oil

½ teaspoon almond oil

1 bar all natural Ivory soap

Craft knife

Parchment paper

Directions:

Soften the bar of soap slight in the microwave. Cut into smaller pieces, and add to a pan on the stove with the coconut and almond oil.

Turn on to medium high heat, and stir often. Let the bar of soap completely melt, and once it has, add in all your essential oils.

Blend well, then remove from heat. Let the mix cool for a while. Stir every few minutes, and once it's cool enough to touch, roll out onto the parchment paper. Use your hands to form into a ball (carefully, you don't want to burn yourself), or use molds.

Let set up for 24 hours, and your handmade soap is done.

Chapter 2 – Little Pampers for Oily Skin

Oily skin or dry skin? Sometimes you have both! With these bars, you are going to get the best of both worlds as you feel moisturized and clean... all at the same time.

The Fair Skinned Princess

What you will need:

15 drops myrrh oil

10 drops ginger oil

5 drops tea tree oil

2 teaspoons coconut oil

½ teaspoon almond oil

1 bar all natural Ivory soap

Craft knife

Parchment paper

Directions:

Soften the bar of soap slight in the microwave. Cut into smaller pieces, and add to a pan on the stove with the coconut and almond oil.

Turn on to medium high heat, and stir often. Let the bar of soap completely melt, and once it has, add in all your essential oils.

Blend well, then remove from heat. Let the mix cool for a while. Stir every few minutes, and once it's cool enough to touch, roll out onto the parchment paper. Use your hands to form into a ball (carefully, you don't want to burn yourself), or use molds.

Let set up for 24 hours, and your handmade soap is done.

The Diva

What you will need:

10 drops jasmine oil

8 drops frankincense oil

8 drops ylang ylang oil

2 teaspoons coconut oil

½ teaspoon almond oil

1 bar all natural Ivory soap

Craft knife

Parchment paper

Directions:

Soften the bar of soap slight in the microwave. Cut into smaller pieces, and add to a pan on the stove with the coconut and almond oil.

Turn on to medium high heat, and stir often. Let the bar of soap completely melt, and once it has, add in all your essential oils.

Blend well, then remove from heat. Let the mix cool for a while. Stir every few minutes, and once it's cool enough to touch, roll out onto the parchment paper. Use your hands to form into a ball (carefully, you don't want to burn yourself), or use molds.

Let set up for 24 hours, and your handmade soap is done.

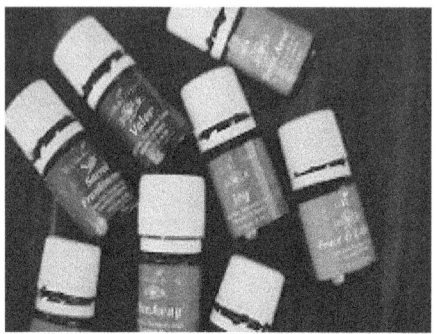

Fairest of Them All

What you will need:

15 drops frankincense oil

5 drops bergamot oil

5 drops geranium oil

2 teaspoons coconut oil

½ teaspoon almond oil

1 bar all natural Ivory soap

Craft knife

Parchment paper

Directions:

Soften the bar of soap slight in the microwave. Cut into smaller pieces, and add to a pan on the stove with the coconut and almond oil.

Turn on to medium high heat, and stir often. Let the bar of soap completely melt, and once it has, add in all your essential oils.

Blend well, then remove from heat. Let the mix cool for a while. Stir every few minutes, and once it's cool enough to touch, roll out onto the parchment paper. Use your hands to form into a ball (carefully, you don't want to burn yourself), or use molds.

Let set up for 24 hours, and your handmade soap is done.

The Swan

What you will need:

18 drops sandalwood oil

10 drops pine oil

3 drops winter green oil

2 teaspoons coconut oil

½ teaspoon almond oil

1 bar all natural Ivory soap

Craft knife

Parchment paper

Directions:

Soften the bar of soap slight in the microwave. Cut into smaller pieces, and add to a pan on the stove with the coconut and almond oil.

Turn on to medium high heat, and stir often. Let the bar of soap completely melt, and once it has, add in all your essential oils.

Blend well, then remove from heat. Let the mix cool for a while. Stir every few minutes, and once it's cool enough to touch, roll out onto the parchment paper. Use your hands to form into a ball (carefully, you don't want to burn yourself), or use molds.

Let set up for 24 hours, and your handmade soap is done.

Luscious Lavender Lilly

What you will need:

15 drops lavender oil

9 drops vetiver oil

8 drops neroli oil

2 teaspoons coconut oil

½ teaspoon almond oil

1 bar all natural Ivory soap

Craft knife

Parchment paper

Directions:

Soften the bar of soap slight in the microwave. Cut into smaller pieces, and add to a pan on the stove with the coconut and almond oil.

Turn on to medium high heat, and stir often. Let the bar of soap completely melt, and once it has, add in all your essential oils.

Blend well, then remove from heat. Let the mix cool for a while. Stir every few minutes, and once it's cool enough to touch, roll out onto the parchment paper. Use your hands to form into a ball (carefully, you don't want to burn yourself), or use molds.

Let set up for 24 hours, and your handmade soap is done.

Chapter 3 – Anti-Aging Soaps and Such

Another year has passed, but no one needs to know what that means for you. With these soaps, you can preserve your natural youth and maintain that captivating aura you have held your entire life.

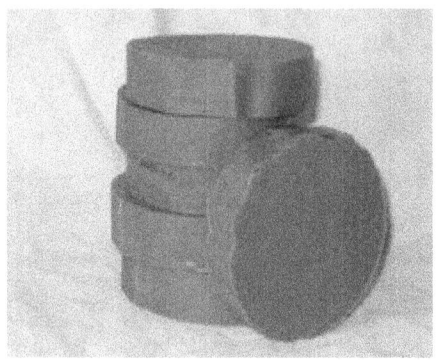

Forever a Queen

What you will need:

15 drops myrrh oil

9 drops Roman chamomile oil

8 drops ylang ylang oil

2 teaspoons coconut oil

½ teaspoon almond oil

1 bar all natural Ivory soap

Craft knife

Parchment paper

Directions:

Soften the bar of soap slight in the microwave. Cut into smaller pieces, and add to a pan on the stove with the coconut and almond oil.

Turn on to medium high heat, and stir often. Let the bar of soap completely melt, and once it has, add in all your essential oils.

Blend well, then remove from heat. Let the mix cool for a while. Stir every few minutes, and once it's cool enough to touch, roll out onto the parchment paper. Use your hands to form into a ball (carefully, you don't want to burn yourself), or use molds.

Let set up for 24 hours, and your handmade soap is done.

Glorious Youth

What you will need:

5 drops tea tree oil

8 drops oregano oil

8 drops spearmint oil

2 teaspoons coconut oil

½ teaspoon almond oil

1 bar all natural Ivory soap

Craft knife

Parchment paper

Directions:

Soften the bar of soap slight in the microwave. Cut into smaller pieces, and add to a pan on the stove with the coconut and almond oil.

Turn on to medium high heat, and stir often. Let the bar of soap completely melt, and once it has, add in all your essential oils.

Blend well, then remove from heat. Let the mix cool for a while. Stir every few minutes, and once it's cool enough to touch, roll out onto the parchment paper. Use your hands to form into a ball (carefully, you don't want to burn yourself), or use molds.

Let set up for 24 hours, and your handmade soap is done.

The Secret Spell

What you will need:

19 drops lemon oil

15 drops lemongrass oil

5 drops orange oil

2 teaspoons coconut oil

½ teaspoon almond oil

1 bar all natural Ivory soap

Craft knife

Parchment paper

Directions:

Soften the bar of soap slight in the microwave. Cut into smaller pieces, and add to a pan on the stove with the coconut and almond oil.

Turn on to medium high heat, and stir often. Let the bar of soap completely melt, and once it has, add in all your essential oils.

Blend well, then remove from heat. Let the mix cool for a while. Stir every few minutes, and once it's cool enough to touch, roll out onto the parchment paper. Use your hands to form into a ball (carefully, you don't want to burn yourself), or use molds.

Let set up for 24 hours, and your handmade soap is done.

The Enchanted Garden

What you will need:

8 drops apple aromatherapy oil

8 drops lavender oil

5 drops cedar oil

2 teaspoons coconut oil

½ teaspoon almond oil

1 bar all natural Ivory soap

Craft knife

Parchment paper

Directions:

Soften the bar of soap slight in the microwave. Cut into smaller pieces, and add to a pan on the stove with the coconut and almond oil.

Turn on to medium high heat, and stir often. Let the bar of soap completely melt, and once it has, add in all your essential oils.

Blend well, then remove from heat. Let the mix cool for a while. Stir every few minutes, and once it's cool enough to touch, roll out onto the parchment paper. Use your hands to form into a ball (carefully, you don't want to burn yourself), or use molds.

Let set up for 24 hours, and your handmade soap is done.

A New Age

What you will need:

8 drops patchouli oil

8 drops blood orange oil

8 drops bergamot oil

2 teaspoons coconut oil

½ teaspoon almond oil

1 bar all natural Ivory soap

Craft knife

Parchment paper

Directions:

Soften the bar of soap slight in the microwave. Cut into smaller pieces, and add to a pan on the stove with the coconut and almond oil.

Turn on to medium high heat, and stir often. Let the bar of soap completely melt, and once it has, add in all your essential oils.

Blend well, then remove from heat. Let the mix cool for a while. Stir every few minutes, and once it's cool enough to touch, roll out onto the parchment paper. Use your hands to form into a ball (carefully, you don't want to burn yourself), or use molds.

Let set up for 24 hours, and your handmade soap is done.

Chapter 4 – Fall Blends

We all look forward to the fall treats that show up year after year. This year, go ahead and indulge in the fall treats... right in your own bathtub. Use as many or as few of the oils as you like, and get the perfect combination, every time.

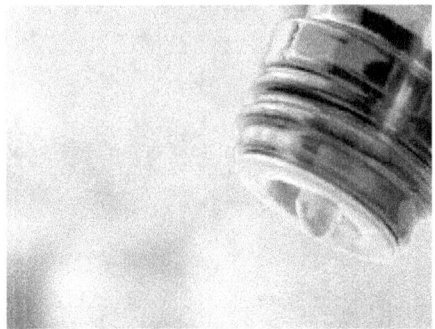

Fall Breeze

What you will need:

10 drops cinnamon oil

5 drops ginger oil

5 drops nutmeg oil

2 teaspoons coconut oil

½ teaspoon almond oil

1 bar all natural Ivory soap

Craft knife

Parchment paper

Directions:

Soften the bar of soap slight in the microwave. Cut into smaller pieces, and add to a pan on the stove with the coconut and almond oil.

Turn on to medium high heat, and stir often. Let the bar of soap completely melt, and once it has, add in all your essential oils.

Blend well, then remove from heat. Let the mix cool for a while. Stir every few minutes, and once it's cool enough to touch, roll out onto the parchment paper. Use your hands to form into a ball (carefully, you don't want to burn yourself), or use molds.

Let set up for 24 hours, and your handmade soap is done.

Autumn Leaves

What you will need:

8 drops cinnamon oil

9 drops vanilla oil

8 drops sandalwood oil

2 teaspoons coconut oil

½ teaspoon almond oil

1 bar all natural Ivory soap

Craft knife

Parchment paper

Directions:

Soften the bar of soap slight in the microwave. Cut into smaller pieces, and add to a pan on the stove with the coconut and almond oil.

Turn on to medium high heat, and stir often. Let the bar of soap completely melt, and once it has, add in all your essential oils.

Blend well, then remove from heat. Let the mix cool for a while. Stir every few minutes, and once it's cool enough to touch, roll out onto the parchment paper. Use your hands to form into a ball (carefully, you don't want to burn yourself), or use molds.

Let set up for 24 hours, and your handmade soap is done.

Sugar and Spice

What you will need:

12 drops cinnamon oil

12 drops vanilla oil

8 drops ginger oil

2 teaspoons coconut oil

½ teaspoon almond oil

1 bar all natural Ivory soap

Craft knife

Parchment paper

Directions:

Soften the bar of soap slight in the microwave. Cut into smaller pieces, and add to a pan on the stove with the coconut and almond oil.

Turn on to medium high heat, and stir often. Let the bar of soap completely melt, and once it has, add in all your essential oils.

Blend well, then remove from heat. Let the mix cool for a while. Stir every few minutes, and once it's cool enough to touch, roll out onto the parchment paper. Use your hands to form into a ball (carefully, you don't want to burn yourself), or use molds.

Let set up for 24 hours, and your handmade soap is done.

Gingerbread House

What you will need:

15 drops ginger oil

8 drops vanilla oil

5 drops myrrh oil

2 teaspoons coconut oil

½ teaspoon almond oil

1 bar all natural Ivory soap

Craft knife

Parchment paper

Directions:

Soften the bar of soap slight in the microwave. Cut into smaller pieces, and add to a pan on the stove with the coconut and almond oil.

Turn on to medium high heat, and stir often. Let the bar of soap completely melt, and once it has, add in all your essential oils.

Blend well, then remove from heat. Let the mix cool for a while. Stir every few minutes, and once it's cool enough to touch, roll out onto the parchment paper. Use your hands to form into a ball (carefully, you don't want to burn yourself), or use molds.

Let set up for 24 hours, and your handmade soap is done.

Baked Goods

What you will need:

12 drops peppermint oil

8 drops cinnamon oil

9 drops vanilla oil

2 teaspoons coconut oil

½ teaspoon almond oil

1 bar all natural Ivory soap

Craft knife

Parchment paper

Directions:

Soften the bar of soap slight in the microwave. Cut into smaller pieces, and add to a pan on the stove with the coconut and almond oil.

Turn on to medium high heat, and stir often. Let the bar of soap completely melt, and once it has, add in all your essential oils.

Blend well, then remove from heat. Let the mix cool for a while. Stir every few minutes, and once it's cool enough to touch, roll out onto the parchment paper. Use your hands to form into a ball (carefully, you don't want to burn yourself), or use molds.

Let set up for 24 hours, and your handmade soap is done.

Chapter 5 – The Holiday Collection

It won't be long before the sounds of Christmas fill the air, and you will want to completely indulge in the season. Now you have the perfect reason to pamper... so go ahead and sing some carols in the shower!

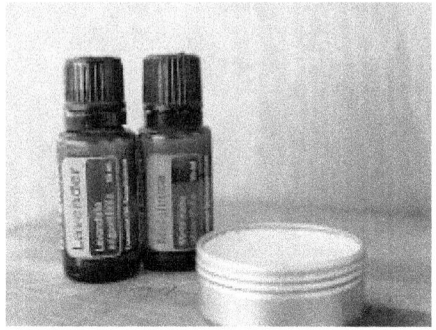

Christmastime Is Here

What you will need:

15 drops winter green oil

10 drops peppermint oil

5 drops pine oil

2 teaspoons coconut oil

½ teaspoon almond oil

1 bar all natural Ivory soap

Craft knife

Parchment paper

Directions:

Soften the bar of soap slight in the microwave. Cut into smaller pieces, and add to a pan on the stove with the coconut and almond oil.

Turn on to medium high heat, and stir often. Let the bar of soap completely melt, and once it has, add in all your essential oils.

Blend well, then remove from heat. Let the mix cool for a while. Stir every few minutes, and once it's cool enough to touch, roll out onto the parchment paper. Use your hands to form into a ball (carefully, you don't want to burn yourself), or use molds.

Let set up for 24 hours, and your handmade soap is done.

Winter Wonder Grand

What you will need:

15 drops peppermint oil

8 drops spearmint oil

2 teaspoons coconut oil

½ teaspoon almond oil

1 bar all natural Ivory soap

Craft knife

Parchment paper

Directions:

Soften the bar of soap slight in the microwave. Cut into smaller pieces, and add to a pan on the stove with the coconut and almond oil.

Turn on to medium high heat, and stir often. Let the bar of soap completely melt, and once it has, add in all your essential oils.

Blend well, then remove from heat. Let the mix cool for a while. Stir every few minutes, and once it's cool enough to touch, roll out onto the parchment paper. Use your hands to form into a ball (carefully, you don't want to burn yourself), or use molds.

Let set up for 24 hours, and your handmade soap is done.

Snowflakes and Lights

What you will need:

15 drops eucalyptus oil

5 drops peppermint oil

5 drops lemon oil

2 teaspoons coconut oil

½ teaspoon almond oil

1 bar all natural Ivory soap

Craft knife

Parchment paper

Directions:

Soften the bar of soap slight in the microwave. Cut into smaller pieces, and add to a pan on the stove with the coconut and almond oil.

Turn on to medium high heat, and stir often. Let the bar of soap completely melt, and once it has, add in all your essential oils.

Blend well, then remove from heat. Let the mix cool for a while. Stir every few minutes, and once it's cool enough to touch, roll out onto the parchment paper. Use your hands to form into a ball (carefully, you don't want to burn yourself), or use molds.

Let set up for 24 hours, and your handmade soap is done.

Spellbound

What you will need:

18 drops myrrh oil

15 drops cedar oil

8 drops pine oil

2 teaspoons coconut oil

½ teaspoon almond oil

1 bar all natural Ivory soap

Craft knife

Parchment paper

Directions:

Soften the bar of soap slight in the microwave. Cut into smaller pieces, and add to a pan on the stove with the coconut and almond oil.

Turn on to medium high heat, and stir often. Let the bar of soap completely melt, and once it has, add in all your essential oils.

Blend well, then remove from heat. Let the mix cool for a while. Stir every few minutes, and once it's cool enough to touch, roll out onto the parchment paper. Use your hands to form into a ball (carefully, you don't want to burn yourself), or use molds.

Let set up for 24 hours, and your handmade soap is done.

Mistletoe Dust

What you will need:

15 drops fir needle oil

10 drops pine oil

8 drops vetiver oil

2 teaspoons coconut oil

½ teaspoon almond oil

1 bar all natural Ivory soap

Craft knife

Parchment paper

Directions:

Soften the bar of soap slight in the microwave. Cut into smaller pieces, and add to a pan on the stove with the coconut and almond oil.

Turn on to medium high heat, and stir often. Let the bar of soap completely melt, and once it has, add in all your essential oils.

Blend well, then remove from heat. Let the mix cool for a while. Stir every few minutes, and once it's cool enough to touch, roll out onto the parchment paper. Use your hands to form into a ball (carefully, you don't want to burn yourself), or use molds.

Let set up for 24 hours, and your handmade soap is done.

Conclusion

There you have it, everything you need to make your own soap and pamper yourself as you deserve to be pampered. I hope this book was able to show you how easy it is to make your own soap, and how you can use the simplest things around you to create the spa of your dreams.

You know you love all the rich scents essential oils give, and when you use them for their benefits, you are going to get more than just a vacation for the senses! Make each of these soaps and discover which is your favorite, and mix and match the recipes for your own creations.

When you are making your own soaps, or any beauty products, you are in complete control. I hope this book was able to show you just how many ways you can modify soaps to be your own, and end up with the perfect bar, every time.

Have fun with the shapes, add food coloring or flower petals for added pampering, and go nuts with the results. When you are in control, you can let your creativity shine in ways you never before could.

So go ahead and grab that bar of soap, you have some modifications to do, and an indulgent bath to take.

FREE Bonus Reminder

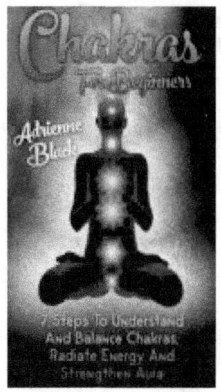

If you have not grabbed it yet, please go ahead and download your special bonus E book *"Chakras for Beginners. 7 Steps To Understand And Balance Chakras, Radiate Energy, And Strengthen Aura"*.

Simply Click the Button Below

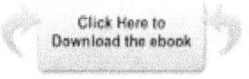

OR Go to This Page

http://lifehacksworld.com/free

BONUS #2: More Free & Discounted Books & Products

Do you want to receive more Free/Discounted Books or Products?

We have a mailing list where we send out our new Books or Products when they go free or with a discount on Amazon. Click on the link below to sign up for Free & Discount Book & Product Promotions.

=> **Sign Up for Free & Discount Book & Product Promotions** <=

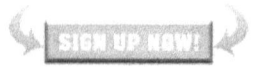

OR Go to this URL

http://zbit.ly/1WBb1Ek

www.ingramcontent.com/pod-product-compliance
Lightning Source LLC
Chambersburg PA
CBHW071309280526
45788CB00004B/1870